BACK TO BASICS
3 STEPS TO
PROFITABLE OPTOMETRY

GORDON DUNCAN

Contents

Copyright 3

Introduction 4

Who are you, anyway? 6
   Teaching 6
   Selling 7
   Eyeballing 8
   Learning From a Consultant 10
   Heading Out on My Own 11
   Consulting on My Own 12

Provide the Best Eye Care 13
   Return to the Optometric Oath 14
   Take Your Time 18
   Hire Quality Staff 23
   Questions 26
   To Sum It Up 29

Keep Costs Low 30
   Don't Overstock 31
   Find Your Price Point 34
   Manage Your Frame Sellers 37
   Questions 40
   To Sum It Up… 43

Increase Revenues 44
   Start at the Front Desk 45
   Convince Them You Care 50
   Spiff Your Staff 52
   Questions 55
   To Sum it Up 58

One Final Note 59

E-books from Gordon Duncan and Jobson Research 60

About the Author 62

Copyright

Copyright © 2016 by Gordon Duncan

All rights reserved. This book or any portion thereof may not be reproduced or used in any manner whatsoever without the express written permission of the author except for the use of brief quotations in a book review.

Published in the United States of America

First Edition, 2016

Introduction

The eye care industry is at a crossroads.

- Government healthcare presents nearly insurmountable challenges.
- Understanding how to code has practically become impossible.
- Costs soar.
- Revenues decrease.
- Quality employees are hard to find.

And the big one…

Few practices make a profit, and even fewer doctors are making a good salary.

This book is here to help. Returning to the basics means returning to the core of what you already know. And it is also enabling you to do the basics so well that you can make money again. So, what are those basics?

1. Provide the best eye care.
2. Keeps costs low.
3. Increase revenues.

That may be as simple as $2 + 2 = 4$. However, ask yourself, "When was the last time I actually did math? Aren't I counting on my phone or calculator to do it?"

Making money in your practice is about returning to the basics of paying attention to the things that you have overlooked or perhaps delegated to someone else.

So, in the following chapters, I am going to give you help to enable you to give the best eye care possible, show you how to lower your costs, and teach you how to increase revenues.

Along the way, I will share real world examples to follow and avoid.

I'm glad you are ready to go back to the basics.

Gordon Duncan
jgordonduncan@gmail.com

Who are you, anyway?

Before we begin looking at the basics, it is important for you to understand who I am, and where I get my philosophy. If you are not interested, then jump ahead to Step One, but I would recommend you read these first pages as they will help you understand how I approach Optometric profitability.

I told my story about how I became an Optometric Consultant in "Practice Progress", but a lot has happened since then. Either way, I enjoy talking about how I arrived to where I am as I hope the story encourages and inspires lots of folks.

If you don't care, that's fine. Just jump on over to the next chapter where we get into the practical, but I do think there is some benefit in this story.

Teaching

I've been a startup/developer for most of my professional life. Graduating from college, I jumped into the world of education where I taught at-risk youth who had already been expelled from grades 6-12. I was fortunate to be a part of an alternative school that sought to lower the drop-out rate in its system. My first day of teaching was the day the school first opened its doors.

During that time, I was immensely blessed to play a part in changing hundreds of students' lives, and I poured every moment of my day into that goal. I wasn't married yet, so my school day rolled into mentoring which then rolled into evenings of study, grading, and lesson planning.

Simultaneously, I had the great benefit of chairing the English Department, designing curriculum, petitioning the credentialing boards to accept our new school, and all of those responsibilities led me to win the school system's Teacher of the Year. I never imagined that, what appeared at first to be a simple teaching job, would give me so many experiences to influence, teach, train, administrate, and understand how to lead and manage people.

I ultimately got married and moved an hour away, so I began to look for a new job. My initial intention was to stay in teaching but only if I could continue in the alternate school structure. The county school system that we moved to didn't have one, so I was left with a choice: teach in the old fashion model or find something new to do.

Selling

One day while playing golf, I received a call from a friend of a friend who was looking for an outside salesperson. While sales was not on my radar, the idea of making enough money to pay off my school loans appealed to me. Working with people who I knew and trusted was important to me as well. I quickly became the salesman for a legal document reproduction company. My job was to convince lawyers and paralegals to trust my company with their confidential documents as they prepared for trial.

All of a sudden, I was cast into a new world where I was still attempting to influence others, but now that sphere involved efficiency (for my staff), profitability (for my boss), and credibility (for my lawyers). I was in charge of gaining new business and taking care of existing clients. I was daily quoting jobs, making promises (that I had to trust others to keep), and knocking on doors to get appointments.

My years in sales taught me great lessons about patience and persistence. Though I was the face of the organization, I could not act alone, and if my support team didn't trust me, they wouldn't perform.

My company eventually decided to open another office out of state. Unfortunately, that office didn't last a single year. My branch was forced to absorb the costs of the failed branch, and I was left answering questions like, "How long can you go without a paycheck?" My answer was, "I don't work for free."

Eyeballing

Perhaps I answered quickly and harshly, but I was not at a place in life where I could just work a month and live without a paycheck. Fortunately, at that same time, an Optometrist friend of mine was in need as his present manager was leaving the workforce to be a full-time mom. After a few meetings, he offered me the job, and I gladly accepted it.

There were some terms of my employment that were key to my taking the job, and as I look back on those things, I can see that my OD did me the biggest favor ever.

In my job, my boss would give me a base salary. He then promised me that he would never give me a raise…ever. However, once I got my legs under me, he would give me 7% of net profit as a bonus. Just for the sake of simplicity. At the end of the month, we looked at how much money we deposited. We would then subtract every penny we spent. If there was anything left over, I got 7% of it.

This was an incredible motivator for me. My doc made it clear: all he wanted to do was come in, turn the dials, and go home. If I was going to be the manager he wanted, then I was going to have to learn and oversee every aspect of the business: front desk, optical, insurance, you name it. If I made those systems work well together, I had the chance to make some real money.

As you can imagine, I cared about every penny, every paperclip, and every patient that walked through the door. We didn't waste anything in that office, and we surely didn't tolerate any one not pulling their weight. Ultimately, I realized that everyone else was going to have to care about the paperclips as well, so I developed a spiff system for the entire office and a specific one for each department. If they cared about the money, then I wouldn't have to worry.

Getting started however, I had to learn the ropes, so I started out by working the front desk for two weeks. I then moved onto pre-testing and optical while my evenings were spent learning how to file insurance and fighting for every dollar. My schooling was quick and overwhelming, but I was soon proficient in each area and my staff learned that I was honest about what I didn't know but confident about what I did. Things rolled along well for several years.

I soon learned that filing insurance for 14,000 patients was too big a job for me to handle in the midst of so many other things, so we farmed it out to a trusted off-site employee. The money spent to file insurance was quickly recouped by the greater percentage of money that was collected.

There were challenges along the way, however. My office was a franchise of a local optometric group. In return for using their software, taking advantage of their discounts, and a few others things, we paid them 4% of billables – that was 4% of what we billed; not 4% of what we collected. I resented writing that check every single month. I just didn't think we received enough benefit for the cost, but that part of the business was a non-negotiable.

Even more annoying to me was the fact that the franchise would send in staff each month to look over our numbers. I will tell you, there is nothing more frustrating than being told how badly you did, especially when you are looking at numbers that you didn't get to see throughout the month. I would be asked why optical sales' averages were dipping or why we didn't see any more patients than we did. Those are difficult questions to answer when you are looking at numbers for the very first time…and they are impossible numbers to change once the month is finished.

My docs would leave those meetings wanting me to do better and work harder. I would leave them frustrated for being the last one in the know.

Ultimately, I made up my mind that I would never go into one of those meetings blindly ever again. I would figure out their systems, determine the numbers myself, and even track them throughout the month so that I could actively affect them. I was done with people yelling at me.

I went home with our monthly numbers printed in detail. I looked at the diagnostics that the franchise honchos cared about and reverse engineered them, and in the process learned their formulas.

I also broke down the prior month's numbers into quarter month increments. I figured out how to project how we were doing with those numbers throughout the month, and I got a better sense for the rhythm of our practice. Next month was going to be different.

As quickly as I learned the numbers and formulas, I taught the staff to do the same. It wasn't going to matter if I cared and they didn't. As they learned how to project and determine the numbers of our days, they grew in working harder towards the things to which they were being held accountable. I soon instituted new financial spiffs for each department. If they hit their numbers, the office hit their numbers, and I hit mine.

I even instituted daily and weekly goals that resulted in food rewards. You won't believe how hard a staff will work for free food. I would say 3-4 out of 5 days, we provided breakfast for the staff, and it was common that we would have lunch on a weekly basis. Often, I would spend a mere $15 on muffins to reward the staff keeping the schedule full. It was pennies spent in return for thousands earned.

Learning From a Consultant

Eventually, one of our contact lens companies gave us a national consultant for an entire week. This is back when the government cared a lot less about gifts from vendors. My consultant was very nice. She figured out that working with me instead of working against me was probably the best plan. She dug into all of our numbers, met with me, the staff, and the doctors, and on her last day, she gave us a giant 3 ring binder of recommendations that we should implement.

She hopped onto her plane, flew away, and left my doctors with the expectation that I was to then put into place everything that she recommended. I had very little time to do any of the things she wanted. I soon found out that our contact lens company spent $5,000 to bring her in for the week. I was stunned and frustrated. Our consultant was nice, but all she did was expect me to change a lot of things that I neither signed off on nor had the time to put into place.

Heading Out on My Own

It was around this time that I started to pursue my Master's degree. My boss told me he didn't care if I took classes as long as it didn't interfere with the profitability of the company. Simultaneously, my doctor sold 51% of the practice to a young OD right out of optometry school. These two decisions (mine and my doctor's) were the beginning of the end for me as a day-to-day manager.

Though my office continued to be profitable at a percentage consistent with my first few years, I was spending less time at the office. Juggling classes and working was hard. I should have handled the whole situation better, but I rationalized my time away by thinking that as long as profits continued, there would not be a conflict.

However, I was not managing our staff as well as I should have been, and my new doctor/owner was not pleased with me at all. He clamped down on my flexible schedule, changed many of the policies, and even proposed changing my bonus structure.

As the majority owner, my new doctor had every right to put whatever policies in place that he wanted. So, he decided to cap my bonuses. He gave me the number and informed that once I received $X amount of bonuses, I wouldn't make any more. Unfortunately, the capping of my bonuses also resulted in the capping of my enthusiasm for my job. Graduate school seemed more and more attractive while the drive to work under the new ownership dimmed. The big questions were:

What am I going to do?
If I quit, how am I going to make a living?
Is it possible to go to school and feed my ever-growing family? (My wife was pregnant with our second daughter.)

One day, after a heated exchange with my doc, which I'm sure was as much my fault as his, I drove to make the bank deposit in an absolute funk. I didn't think that I could keep up the miserable existence that was managing the office. I'm sure the doctors wanted me to leave as much as I wanted to leave.

I called my wife that day, and said, "Honey, I think I'm going to put in a 4 month notice today. That will give me time to train someone to take my place and give me time to figure out how we are going to make a living." In an incredible sign of trust, my remarkable wife agreed with me and encouraged me to do just that.

My doctor gladly accepted my offer. That was the easy part. Now, how in the world was I going to keep a roof over my family's house while finishing school?

Consulting on My Own

Since those fateful days over ten years ago, I have been an Optometric Consultant. I have worked with over fifty docs in multiple states, written several books on everything from Optometry to small business, and I have even started two churches. I love what I do.

I've worked with the one doctor shop with just one other employee. And, I've worked with the doc who owns multiple sites in multiple towns. I've worked with moldy, dusty storefronts, and I've worked with doctors with brand new facilities. I've worked with docs who couldn't tell you how much money was in the bank, and I've worked with docs who knew the exact penny. I've worked with docs who were barely making it day to day, and I've worked with docs who were banking tons of cash.

The stories of these practices that I have worked with will pop up as we move forward, but what I hope for you is to find just that: hope.

I want you to have hope each day as you walk into your practice. I'm not going to assume who you are. You might be the owner, you might be the manager, you might be a hired doc, or you might be the person answering the phone. Either way, I'm going to talk about how your practice can continue, can adapt, and can grow.

So, towards that end, let's get back to the basics. The first step to returning to the basics is Providing the Best Eye Care. Let's jump in.

Provide the Best Eye Care

Do you remember the foundation of your Optometric training?
Do you remember the excitement of learning?
Do you remember the dreams you had when you graduated from Optometry School?

How are you doing in meeting them?

Every doctor that I have worked with started with a great desire to care for patients.

Some have wanted to prevent diseases like glaucoma.
Some have wanted to help children see better.
Some have wanted to help athletes.
Some doctors went years without proper eye care and wanted to make sure that no one went through that ever again.

And most want to make a good living, and there is nothing wrong with that.

So, you launched into Optometry School. You risked a ton. Perhaps you took on some debt. You asked your parents to support you a bit longer.

I know OD's who waited to have children just so they could finish school. You know what great sacrifice is.

So, to return you to the heights of quality care that you aspired to, let's approach it this way. To provide quality eye care, let's…

Return to the Optometric Oath
Take Your Time
Hire Quality Staff

Return to the Optometric Oath

Now one of the things, that either your school or your state board, demanded of you was adherence to the Optometric Oath

Do you remember the Optometric Oath? As a reminder, let's walk through it. And as we do, it will be the first path towards profitability and providing quality eye care.

With full deliberation I freely and solemnly pledge that: I will practice the art and science of optometry faithfully and conscientiously, and to the fullest scope of my competence.

Those are lofty goals. They are also even more lofty promises. Now, before we take it step by step, ask yourselves these questions:

When did you first read that oath?
When did you take it?
Do you think about regularly?
Do you seek to live it out each day in your practice?

To answer those last questions, let's look at the oath bit by bit.

With full deliberation

This means you thought through taking the oath before you made it. You weighed whether it was true, and youed look at your character to see if the oath was consistent with who you are.

I solemnly pledge

Pretty close to swearing in court or in a marriage vow, isn't it? A vow is a vow.

I will practice

This is practice like an athlete. Practice in this sense means that you will pursue your craft as a profession with the goal of acquiring skill and proficiency.

The art and science of optometry

What you do is not a hobby or a proclivity. You are an artist, a scientist.

Faithfully and conscientiously

You are consistent and aware of doing a good job each and every day.

And to the fullest scope of my competence

You care for patients to the extent your license allows to the extent your skill enables.

That's a lot to take in again, isn't it?

It's been awhile since you thought about those things I bet. But getting back to the basics starts with providing the best eye care to which you are able.

You may make quick money at a slash and burn/prescribe eyeglasses hut, but those practices will neither give you nor a profitable income. To enjoy what you do and make money, you have to be a good Optometrist, period. I've never met a hack eye doctor who enjoys what he/she does and make money (at least not for the long run).

Let me tell you a story.

I consulted with a doctor in a semi-rural town for several years. And though once skilled, he was distracted.

His hobbies took precedent.
Home was an afterthought.
And he only saw his practice as a means to pursue his hobbies and to keep his family demands at bay.

What was the result?

He came in late.
He gave quick eye exams.
He was over demanding of his staff.
He was under demanding of himself.
And he was generally annoyed with having to show up in the first place.

His practice's problems were myriad. However, none of them were going to change in any positive direction until he took his profession more serious.

His practice was, by all means, an afterthought.

His family knew that he didn't care.
His staff knew that he didn't care.
His patients knew that he didn't care.

In all accounts, he was a hacky eye doctor who gave sub-standard care.

As a consultant, I'm rarely asked to address a doctor's personal issues. Those needs were beyond my scope both professionally and personally. But his practice was my scope.

After working with him for a period of time, I found that his A/R was a mess. His inventory was over-stuffed. His staff was grumpy and overpaid.

Basically every issue imaginable.

But I tackled the hard one – the one that he didn't want to address. One day at lunch, I told him that I didn't think he was taking his practice seriously.

I told him that he wasn't taking his profession seriously.
Oh, I could motivate staff.
I could give them bonus opportunities.
I could clean up the optical inventory.
I could train his insurance person.

That day at lunch, I told him that all of those things were being addressed. But until he found a desire to practice again, no real change would occur. In fact, until he found a desire to practice full-scope optometry faithfully and conscientiously, no real change would occur.

He didn't. His practice didn't improve. If it is still in business, I would be surprised.

My hope when you hear this story is that you care so much about being an eye care professional that you think I wouldn't have to make that assessment about you.

In fact, I hope that you are such a professional that you would be offended if I said that about you. If that is the case, you are on the right track.

But unfortunately, being a quality eye doctor is not all that is necessary any more.

There are so many mega-chains right now
Each of them could easily swallow you or be swallowed up.
They either want to buy you out or push you out.
Healthcare reimbursement is at an all-time low.
The cost of doing business is rising.

But before addressing these issues, ask yourself, "Am I faithfully and conscientiously practicing the art and science of optometry?" If that answer is not an unequivocal "yes", then let's start there.

Even if you can say "yes" without hesitation, I still think there are areas, blind spots, that you can address that will enable you to enjoy practicing and make more money.

Towards that end, let's look at our second reminder to provide quality eye care.

Take Your Time

The first step to providing quality eye care is taking your time.

Hear me out. I'll be the first one to tell you that if you can do three quality, comprehensive eye exams in an hour, do them. See three an hour as many hours per days as you can. Full eye-exams drive your revenue.

But, don't make your patients feel like they are in an assembly line.

You know this. You know that no one wants to feel like they are being rushed…especially in a medical scenario.

Storytime

Recently, my family relocated. In our prior home, I had a choice of a dozen eye doctors who would give me and my family eye exams – most of which would be free because of my prior experience with helping them with their practices. So, I had the privilege of choosing the O.D. I thought was best. I didn't have to worry about money, insurance, or anything else. I was thankful…and picky.

But in our new state, I was looking for an eye doctor like all of your patients. On top of all of that, we also had new insurance. Since it was taken by one of the new mega-chains, I thought I would check out one of their newly purchased practices.

I knew their inner workings a bit because one of the doctors who I consulted with asked me to walk them through an acquisition by them. But I was incredibly curious about what it was like to be a patient.

My wife was the guinea pig. She was the one who needed the exam, so she set an appointment. I gladly tagged along and never mentioned that I was a consultant.

First, their processes were very tight and smart. They didn't miss a chance to greet us well and to offer us opportunities to maximize revenue (all of that I am for and support).

But the second point was the concern. The time with the O.D. was cold, quick, and overly efficient. Neither one of us wanted to ever see her again.

Again, maximize your time, but give the patient as much time as needed. That was something that my wife never received. The entire time, the O.D. gave the impression that she was setting her up to just move on to the next room.

Her questions were cold and quick.
There was little to no personal interaction.
She gave the impression that all she cared about was selling year's supplies and a new pair of glasses.

Again, I will tell you to sell a year's supplies of contact lenses and new glasses, but if you do that at the sacrifice of your patient's knowing you personally, you will either lose them as patients or your practice will eventually suffer.

You may hear my example and think, "Well, that was just one day. That was just one doctor. Everyone has a bad day."

Well, I actually gave that chain another opportunity a few months later.

Same chain.
Different doctor.
Same deal.
Same rush job.
Same impersonal interaction.

In fact, in following up with the O.D. I know in the chain, he said the chain's internal diagnostics value contact lenses sells over patient satisfaction and patient retention.

Think about that. The company's internal diagnostics weight contact lens sells over patient satisfaction and patient retention.

Back to the Basics
3 Steps to Profitable Optometry
Gordon Duncan

That's a quick grab with a short sight for the future.

But, what if you could do both?
What if you could care about patient satisfaction and revenue?
What if patients left your exam room knowing that you gave them your full attention?

Let's walk through this simple exercise to move you there.

I'm a new patient to your practice. I present with a fairly simple script. I have a bit of a stigmatism, don't really care for contacts, and my glasses are only about two years old. I'm wearing cargo shorts, running shoes, and a YMCA shirt (which is pretty much what I wear unless I am consulting with you).

Your tech has me set in the chair.
My health history and medicine profile is complete and is set in the computer.
My pressures have been tested and documented.
Autorefractor and corneal curvatures have done their job.
The phoropter is set to my RX.

With so many things done for you, an eye exam with no issues presenting can be done in less than 10 minutes. I bet you could do it in 6 or 7 minutes.

But that's not the point is it?

You want your tech to put you in this place, correct?
You want your tech to set you up for an efficient exam, right?
Efficiency says, "Let the tech do everything they can do. The doctor should do the things that only doctors do."

But 6 or 7 minutes is not going to gain you loyal patients – not when the patient gets the overwhelming amount of their time with your front desk person, tech, and framer seller. (By the way, those 3 better be incredible. That is a topic for another paragraph.) And to be honest, you are only going to get as much as 9 or 10 if you are working on a 15 minute exam schedule.

Well, first of all. You can do stuff like the cover test, the refraction, and slit-lamp exam in your sleep. You've done them a thousand times. But remind yourself. Doing things that you've done a thousand times means you can do them well. The athlete at the free throw line can take the shot well because they have practiced free throws in the gym over and over again, but they make the shot when they take their time.

If you rush even what you know how to do well, you are not going to do it well.

And your patients will notice.

But a quality eye exam that shows your patients that you care is not about adding another minute or even adding 30 seconds. A quality eye exam that shows your patients that you care is about what you do in that minute or 30 seconds.

So, let's be hokie, cheesy or whatever you want to call it.

Here it is. Here is how taking your time will make you a more profitable practice.

Spend time with your patients.
Get to know them.
Talk to them about their kids.
Care for them.

If you take the full amount of time that you can to give quality exam AND you interact with your patients, you will become a more profitable practice.

Listen, you know which patients of yours just want to get in and get out. Let them. Scoot them along.

But the patients who want to get time with you, give it. If you make them feel comfortable, if you let them know that you genuinely care about them...

They will be more willing to spend their money with you.
They will be more loyal.
They will tell their friends about you.

Why? Because they like you. They believe you care about them. They think you are in this for more than money.

You see the irony, right?

You don't spend time with them merely to get them to spend more money. But if you spend time with them, they will spend more money.

No matter, what the most ardent penny-pincher tries to do, they still are loyal to good care. If you care for them, not just their eyes, but really care for them, then you will become a more profitable eye care provider.

Take your time during the exam.
Take time getting to know your patient, or getting to know them better.
And your practice will grow in most every way.

Hire Quality Staff

Of course every doctor knows to hire quality staff, right?
No one needs to teach that, right?
Sure every office is filled with amazing staff, right?

But you know this is not the case. After working with dozens of doctors, I promise you I know this is not the case.

So, why is it, when we know that hiring quality staff will provide the best eye care possible, that our offices are full of sub-standard, cranky, hard to take directions, staff?

I'll offer a couple of suggestions. Let's start with the one I find most often in doctor's offices.

You don't like firing people.

I cannot tell you how many times doctors allow terrible employees to continue working for them. After a while, I just ask them, "Why haven't you fired them? Why are they still working here?"

And the answer is something like, "I just don't like firing them."

Sometimes, there is an answer like, "You don't know how long they've worked here."

Or, "Oh man, she just had a baby."

Granted, I understand those reasons are challenging. Most people don't like putting people out of a job. And people who have worked for you, or your office for 10+ years are more difficult to fire. And most employees are dependent upon the paycheck you give them.

But, terrible employees are killing your practice.

They cause patients to schedule their exam somewhere else.
They cause patients to buy their materials somewhere else.
They cause patients to tell other potential patients to go somewhere else.

And you know the rule. Disgruntled patients will tell 10 friends if they don't like your practice.

And if you are depositing $300 or more per patient, and I hope you do, then that patient plus those 10 friends are going to cost you $3,330 (the first year).

And none of this even includes future income lost.

That is the cost of your not liking to fire bad employees.

You hire family or friends.

Please, oh please don't hire family or friends.

Don't get me wrong. I have seen family and friends function well in an office environment, but more times than not, it goes poorly. Family and friends performing well in an office are the exception and not the rule.

Here is why…

Most of the time, a doctor struggles to manage, much less reprimand, friends and relatives. It's okay. You are a good person. You don't want to damage your relationship with your spouse or your buddy by telling them they aren't doing a good job. It's hard to tell your spouse, "Hey, if you don't start showing up on time, you can't really tell everyone else they have to show up on time." That will make for an awkward evening.

Additionally, the terrible habit that I see doctors falling into is hiring under-gifted friends and over-paying them. They do this because they feel like they can trust them, but let's be honest. Almost no employee is worth hiring and overpaying if they don't have the skills (and on a side note, this will embitter your employees, especially your talented ones).

The easy rule is this: Do not hire anyone that you are not willing to fire.

And if you are convinced you would be willing to fire anybody who underperforms, check yourself this way. Hire them only with a 90 day probation period. This will show you whether they are willing to be an employee under your leadership and discretion.

Granted, some of you are in situations that you may not be able to get out of (i.e. firing your wife). But going forward, just avoid anybody that would cause you angst to fire.

You don't hire quality people in the first place.

This is the best time in the world to hire people. Despite the impression, there are tons of quality, potential employees out there. It takes time and a ton of effort. If you don't give hiring the time it deserves, your patients won't get the care they need.

And we know, if the patients don't get the care they need, they go somewhere else and tell everyone else how bad their experience was.

Listen, I've hired lots of employees with varied backgrounds, and many who knew next to nothing about optometry. But the ones I've hired like that had crazy people skills, and I didn't put them in a technical area.

Read: They were trainable, and they weren't in over their heads.

It is better for you to leave a position open than to fill it with an employee who doesn't have the personality or skill set to properly care for you patients.

Questions

(The intention of this book is to provide a small space to work through these questions. So, if you happen to be reading this in e-from, feel free to print these pages or email me at jgordonduncan@gmail.com, and I'll get them to you.)

Do you remember when you first read the Optometric Oath? Did you weigh what you were reading and vowing? How are you doing with keeping up your promises?

If a stranger asked you how Optometry was an "art and science", how would you answer it? How do you practice it as an art and science?

What about your practice is full scope Optometry?

Do you think you take your time during your eye exams? Why or why not?

Against what do you measure "taking your time"? Time your actual time in the room with your patients. Just click the timer on your phone on the way in, and click it again on the way out. Do you think that is sufficient to provide quality eye care? Why or why not?

Is your staff quality? Again, how do you measure quality?

Is there another doctor in your area that you think has a more quality staff? What makes them better?

Is there a staff member that you keep around only because you don't want to fire them? What's keeping you from letting poor staff go?

What is preventing you from hiring more quality employees?

To Sum It Up

So, that's the first step.

If you want to get back to the basics of being a profitable doctor and practice, you have to provide quality eye care.

If you begin to take your time and hire quality staff, you will put yourself in place to either move towards profitability or to grow your profits.

Having said that, let's move on to step 2.

Keep Costs Low

I'll be the first to agree with the axiom: to make money, you have to spend money. However, and this is important, make sure that every penny you spend is worth it.

If you only spend money that's worth spending, then your costs will be low in comparison to your deposits. Appropriate costs in relation to deposits equal substantial profits.

So, let's figure out how to do that. I will offer these tips to keeping your costs low:

Don't Overstock
Find Your Price Point
Manage Your Frame Sellers

Now, before we start, let me caution you. Almost every single doctor that I have ever met is sure that they have a good hold of their inventory. When I ask them how they know, they typically speak of a trustworthy employee who they have in charge of their frames.

Again, countless numbers of times, said trusted employee cannot tell me either how many frames they have or what the value of the frames are. Heck, they often can't even tell me how many they sell on average each month or how many they need to sell to justify the frames they carry.

These are answers that need to be known so that they can be managed.

So, towards that end, let's take our first tip to keep costs down: don't overstock.

Don't Overstock

How many frames does your office have on the boards?
How many are counted as "understock" – frames off the board?
What is the total value of all frames on hand?
How many frames does your office sell per day, week, and month?

These are just a few of the questions that need answers as you, or your employee, manage your frame stock. No matter what, don't overstock.

Now, why in the world would an office carry too many frames?

The simplest answer is your frame buyer purchases what he/she likes (on your dollar) and doesn't keep track of what is in understock. Seriously, does your frame seller know what you have in stock? Would they not buy some frames if they knew how many they had...even if it was a "good deal"?

Let me tell you a story.

I began working with an Optometrist who owned a large practice in a rural town. Despite the town's size, he had built a huge practice rivaling the size of many metropolitan practices with which I had worked.

But the story was the same. Once I got in there, I discovered that he had almost nothing in the bank.

How could this be? Especially, when you are the number one doc in town?

There were many answers to that question (high patient A/R, high insurance A/R, uncollected co-pays, etc). But one issue predominated...understock.

This doc had a crazy high cost of goods because there were over 1,000 frames in understock. We did a quick estimate. At $59 to $79 per frame (yes, he paid that much), the math was easy. This doctor had $59,000 to $79,000 worth of frames sitting around and gathering dust. In fact, some of them were so old, they would either never sell or they would have to sell for $29 or something terrible like that.

You can't keep your costs low if what you are buying is useless, tucked into boxes, and forgotten. The only purpose of your understock is to support your frame board. That's it.

So, that leads us to this question:

How many frames should you carry on your frame board?

I would suggest whatever you can turn over 2.5 times a year. This is the industry standard and for good reason. If you sell 1,000 frames a year (God bless you by the way), then you need 400 frames on your board. Along the way, you don't really need any more than about 50 frames in understock.

If your attempt is to carry every size and every color of every frame, then you are going to go broke, so don't try to do it.

There is another distinct advantage to carrying the number of frames that you can turn over 2.5 times (in addition to the cost savings). That number of frames keeps the patient from being overwhelmed, and an overwhelmed patient goes elsewhere. Let me explain.

When you go to a car dealer, they set the cars up in an attractive way to get your attention. You'll find a couple of high end, exclusive cars in the showroom. A few other cars will be in prominent display out in front. You might find 2-3 rows of cars on each side, and not much else. Now, there are a ton more cars out back, but everything is set out in such a way that the buyer is not overwhelmed. If you want a certain color or a certain option, they go and find the car for you on the lot or call another dealership in town. But what you see is just enough to entice you.

Though this is an imperfect analogy, I think you see where I'm going. If you sell 1,000 frames a year, and they are all on the board, the patient can't see the forest for the trees. The dealer doesn't put every car they are going to sell on the lot at the same time and they strategically place the ones available just in sight.

Even Wal-Mart opticals don't put every frame out. They have a ton of understock because they can afford it, but they are very specific and choosy about what makes it onto the board. Everything at one time is just too much.

So don't put a ton of frames on your board. Too many options equals too many decisions which just might result in no sale for you.

Find Your Price Point

I may very well write this in every book that I write.

Are you ready? Okay, here it goes.

You cannot compete with Wal-Mart

Here is what I mean. If you think $79 for a full set of glasses or making your living off of cheap "Buy one; get one free" offers is going to help you compete against the world's largest company (and 25th largest national economy), then you are fooling yourself. Wal-Mart could pay every independent OD's patients to leave their practices, give them a set of frames in their store, and still make money. So, when you choose to stock your board, you have to take a couple of approaches.

First of all, you don't have to be a boutique ($300 frames and up only), but if you can be, go for it. If not a boutique, at least act like one.

Let me explain. If you try to make a living in the "buy one get one free" world, you lose the right to be critical of massive chains. To sell "buy one get one", you have to sell cheap frames. You can't point out their (quite often) inferior quality if you are doing the exact same thing. They can at least afford to replace junk frames that break, and you can't. Aim higher.

If someone asks you if you have special deals or $79 full sets, offer this advice to them.

"While I respect my other OD's who work at Wal-Mart, the reason those frames are so cheap is because they are inferior quality. I never want one of my patients to walk out the door only to have them return a month later with frames that fell apart in their hands."

In terms of the economy, address it in this way.

"I know that paying a couple of hundred dollars for a pair of glasses is not easy these days. But what is even worse is spending money on an inferior pair of glasses that is going to waste your time and cause you to make multiple trips to Wal-Mart. And you know what that optician is going to do? They'll offer to replace it no problem, and then they'll suggest you walk around Wal-Mart in the meantime. You'll get another set of junk glasses, and you can pick them up right after you spend $100 in the super store."

I'm not joking. Be that honest. Sell quality frames and make no excuses for either their cost or their quality. Trust me on this. I would rather go broke selling quality materials than go broke replacing junk frames and having really expensive employees waste time doing the same thing over and over again.

Sell quality. Sell service. Sell what you can offer that they can't: personal service that is second to none.

So, what do you charge for your frames? Well, here is what most docs do. They have a set mark up for their frames. I know some that double and some that triple their frame cost. I recommend tripling, but look at your market and make your determination. But don't stop there. If all you do is triple your frame cost, then you have a million different prices on your board. That doesn't help sales. Let me explain.

When a patient looks at your board and they find every frame has a different price, two things stick in their mind: the highest and lowest price. The highest price is probably beyond their budget, so their mind settles on the lower number. Let's say that number is $99. They are going to go cheapest, but they are probably going to stay somewhere around that number. So what do you do?

The answer is set price points and stick to them in your optical. Here is the concept. Set your cheapest frame price. I would suggest $99, but if you feel like you have to go to $79, do that. Then set your highest frame price say at $399. Then determine 5 prices in between that are equal amounts apart. For example, your board prices would look like this.

$99, $159, $219, $279, $339, and $399

Some folks like to do away with all their frames ending in 9, but that is probably neither here nor there. The idea with price points works like this. You want repetitive prices sticking in your patient's head. When they see the same number come up again and again, most patients will kick out the highest and lowest and settle on a good number in between. If you have 400 frames and 400 frame prices, the patient's mind sticks to the highest and the lowest.

So when you get your frames in, pricing is easy. The formula will look like this. And again, I'll use the 3x's mark up as our example.

Frame Cost x 3 rounded up to the closest price point.

So, if you buy a lot of frames for $66 dollars, then this is how you will price them. $66 x 3 = $198. Then you round it up to $219. If you get frames at a special rate, still use the standard frame cost for that frame. So if you buy lot of frames that are typically $99 at the price of $79, use the $99 cost. $99 frames x 3 = $297. You'll round those frames up to $339.

Then, you'll be keeping your prices down and profits up.

In the end, you may decide that price points are not the way to go. That's fine, but I will encourage you to resist an infinite number of frame prices. No matter what, just make the pricing of your frames strategic. If this system doesn't work, so be it. Either find another or create your own, but don't let that revenue stream go un-shepherded.

Manage Your Frame Sellers

How this became a problem is the same way to fix it.

First, put this rule in place.

You are the final frame buyer.

That doesn't mean you have to approve every frame that is purchased. It means you need parameters. We covered some of these topics in "Practice Progress", so I won't go into them as deeply, but there are a few points that bear repeating.

Remember again: you are the final frame buyer. I don't care how great your seller/optician is, give them a financial limit. Tell them they have the freedom to buy frames to a certain dollar amount or to a certain number, but any potential purchase that exceeds those amounts has to be approved by you.

When I managed an office, I used to tell my optical folks this second truth all the time, but they always struggled to believe it.

The frame vendor is not your friend.

What I mean is that they are not your personal friend. Oh, they might take you out to eat, and I've even known a few to show up at birthday parties and the like, but the end goal of that frame vendor is to make the sale.

I've seen offices that gave frame vendors nearly 100% freedom to bring in frames, which is insane – not your employees, but frame vendors. If you give a salesperson unrestrained freedom, what you are going to get is an unrestrained frame bill. And don't let the vendor fool you with the old "I'm just going to swap out some frames" routine. If you don't know what I'm talking about, let me explain with this scenario.

Your optical person tells the frame vendor that you won't be buying any new frames from them this visit. They respond with, "Hey, no problem. Everyone is tightening up right now. I'll help you out and take some of these old frames that aren't selling and just put some new one out to help boost your sales. We'll just swap out the old ones for new ones."

Then guess what happens?

You get a bill for $500.

I'm not impugning every vendor. Some of them have amazing integrity, but their job is to make the sale. They make more money the more frames that they sell. Whenever a vendor wants to "swap out" here is the simple rule.

Tell them that if they want to take away frames that aren't selling and replace them with newer frames, that is great. But in the end, the effect on your account must either be that I have a credit for returned frames or the swap out costs me nothing. Period.

Any vendor that violates this rule or this trust will be placed on probation or banned. It may sound harsh, but no vendor has your interests first. Only you do.

Once I put this rule in place, I faced a ton of opposition from my optical staff. They said our vendors were honest and that it would damage our relationships with them if we started talking to them that way. I asked them what some of our vendors had done for them lately in terms of gifts and meals. They listed a string of gifts. That was the real problem. They didn't want to lose all their freebies, but the problem was that their freebies came at a cost of thousands of dollars to the office.

What you'll find with this approach is that you'll be offered a lot less swapping deals, but if you do, you'll get new frames at no additional cost.

Do not be swayed on this.
Implement this policy now.
Do not be dissuaded by your optical staff.

If you don't manage or restrain your optical folks from buying, you are going to wind up with a ton of understock. And if you manage, or eliminate, that understock, you will keep your costs low.

Lower costs equal higher profits.

And by managing your understock, demanding that all swap-outs be new product with no additional cost, you will also keep frame selection fresh without spending any extra money.

Questions

Do you know what your inventory costs are in your practice? Why or why not? What are they?

Are your inventory costs proportionate to your revenue? How so?

Who has the last say to purchase frames in your practice? Does that need to be modified?

How much understock do you have? Get someone to give you an exact count and value. Adjust accordingly.

Do you turn your frame boards over 2.5 times a year? Why or why not? If you turn it over 3 times a year, you may not carry enough stock. If you turn it over less than 2 times a year, you have too much.

Do you use price points? If you don't, how does your practice determine the price of your frames?

If you don't determine the price of your frames, spend time with your frame seller asking him or her how they do it.

How are your frames grouped in your frame room? Design a flow for your patients so that they don't wander aimlessly through the room.

To Sum It Up...

Low costs don't happen in a practice by accident. They happen strategically and by your choice.

And while the oversight recommended here may seem like more work for you, it won't be in the long run. Once you establish these new practices, your frame sellers will either improve or be replaced. Either way, these disciplines will establish a cost-effective practice for your frame room.

But here is the thing. No matter how great your frame seller is, you cannot leave them alone forever. Monthly, or at least, quarterly check ups will keep them accountable. And we'll talk next chapter about keeping them motivating.

But know this, if you keep your costs low, you will quickly be on your way to greater profits. Now, let's look at the third step...

Increase Revenues

Ahh, the age old question: How do I increase revenue?

Well, let's start with this. You can increase revenue all you want, and if you haven't started providing the best eye care and keeping your costs low, it won't matter. You won't be profitable.

Make all the money you want, but you will give it all away to either escalating costs or decreasing patient load unless you start squaring up steps 1 and 2.

Seriously. How frustrating will it be to put more money in the bank just to watch more of it go out? It is time your practice started serving you.

And let me say this as we go forward, this chapter is not about patient acquisition. You know the routes: social media, chamber of commerce, rest homes. What I'm going to help you do is increase revenue with the patients you have. So, acquiring patients is a book for another day.

Having said that, let's make some money. If you want to increase revenue, you need to do 3 things.

Start With the Front Desk
Convince Them You Care
Spiff Your Staff

Start at the Front Desk

I can't remind you enough to hire good employees. Let's be honest, if your front desk person doesn't greet people with a smile and answer the phone with a smile, then you should fire them.

What do you see a day? 10 comprehensive exams? 20? 25?

Watch them go away to another doctor or spend less money when they are with you if you have a less than pleasant front-desk person.

A smile for a front desk person is like good hands for a wide receiver and the ability to sew for a designer. I'll go even further. A chef who can't cook is as good as a front desk person with no smile.

Again, no manner of loyalty or experience is worth keeping a front desk person around who can't smile. And don't even get me started about how unpleasant it must be for your staff to be around them.

Okay, get me started.

An irritable front desk person creates an unhappy staff.
An unhappy staff is an unmotivated staff.
An unmotivated staff does not care for patients well.
And if you don't care for patients, you can forget increasing revenue.

But enough about your front desk person's smile. Let's assume you have the sweetest, kindest front desk person or you are about to hire one. How are they going to help you increase revenue?

Let me give you a list.

The front desk takes insurance information. No insurance info means you don't get paid.

The front desk schedules your appointments. What if they like to keep Fridays light so they can get off on time?

The front desk handles every insurance question on the front end. What if they don't explain well why they have to pay for the contact lens exam?

The front desk checks every single person out. What if they can't explain the difference between an insurance frame allowance and an insurance discount?

The front desk pulls every chart/e-record for every patient. What if they aren't ready when the patient walks in? They need to have them ready in the morning and recheck again mid-day. Additionally, they need to check them at the end of the day to make sure they are ready for opening up.

Here are a few more front-desk profit points…

Your front desk must make sure every patient understand that all co-pays are due at time of service.

Your front desk needs to be able to explain contact lens' fees to patients.

Your front desk needs to help your patients understand that they can neither order contacts nor receive a copy of their prescription unless they have paid for the contact lens services.

Your front desk must have a zero tolerance policy in terms of allowing patients to leave with outstanding balances.

Your front desk must never schedule new services or order new product if they have an outstanding balance.

Your front desk must be well-versed in making sure that patients understand all services are paid at the time of service.

Your front desk person is the entry point and exit point for increasing your profit. They must be the utmost professionals in your practice.

Story Time...

I worked for an office who had a better than average front desk person. She answered the phone and greeted people with a smile. She was a bit slow on the computer, but she was a good enough front desk person to keep.

But...she came in late 5-7 minutes every day.

She felt like it was no big deal because she was a good employee. But, it was a big deal. The other employees had to check patients in when she wasn't there, and her tardiness drove the doctors crazy. They spoke to her about it over and over again. It would get better, but then she would fall right back into her old habits...blaming traffic, alarm clocks, and everything else.

One day, she came in her usual 7 minutes late...with a McDonald's cup of coffee in her hand. Usually, this is the kind of stuff that the doctor and the staff put up with. Why not? They put up with it almost every day.

But this day was different. The other employees weren't there to cover for her in those 7 minutes. They weren't supposed to anyway. They were supposed to come in 30 minutes after her, but they came in early most days because they were good, conscientious employees.

So, she walks in 7 minutes late with coffee in hand. But this day, not one, but two patients were at the door, waiting to be checked in for their appointment. And they let her have it. She was late opening the doors with a cup of coffee in her hand. Those 2 patients were so mad, they complained long enough for the next patient to show up. Now, nearly the doctor's first hour of exams was witnessing this mess...all over a cup of coffee.

The doctor lost at least 2 patients that day who faithfully came in every year. The calculated cost of that, conservatively, is $12,000 over the lifetime of the patient. They each averaged $300 of revenue each year times 20 more visits. So, they lost $600 times 20. That number might be higher because we have no idea how many people they told about their miserable service.

Now, the doctor didn't fire her then and there. He was fearful about the fallout since he had tolerated her tardiness to that point.

So I stepped in. The doctor needed a solution. He needed her to improve drastically before they lost any more patients or he needed just cause to fire her.

So, I put a probationary plan in place (something I recommend for any employee you are having trouble reforming). I sat down with her face to face with a written explanation of her tendencies to arrive late. I also pulled her time sheet and logged how many times that she had been tardy.

Recognizing that the doctor had tolerated her lateness, I expressed in both written form and verbally what was expected. For the next 90 days, if she came in late 3 times, she would be fired. 3 times were allowed for things like traffic and other providential hindrances. The employee had two choices with the probation. She could agree to it or quit. Her agreement required her to sign the probationary agreement. She kept a copy, and we put a copy in her employee file.

Believe it or not, she made it 90 days and was only late once. The moment that 90 days was up, we had a staff meeting with an amendment to the employee handbook. It stated that any employee who was late more than 3 times over a 90 period would be terminated.

That's right. The probationary period became standard for the office. Terrible employees weeded themselves out. Good employees kept their job.
The front desk is the person that handles most everything in the front and back end of the office. While every employee needs to be coached and managed, you cannot get away with a poor front desk person.

Now, before we wrap this section up, let me give you a list of things to keep an eye out for your front desk person. In no particular order, your front desk person needs to excel in these areas…

Patient hand off to your patient tech.
Engaging with patients while they wait.
Proper explanation to patients if the doctor is running late.
Never speak authoritatively in areas beyond the front desk's responsibility.
Never diagnose anyone.
Speak sympathetically when scheduling a patient who has a long wait for the next available exam.
Never promise that any insurance company is going to do anything for a patient.
Properly explain all the details of their invoice and billing.

While a detailed book about each area of your office is probably necessary (maybe that one's next), the profitable practice must start at the front desk person. Big or small, every practice has one. Handle well, and watch your profit increase.

With that area covered, let's move on to…

Convince Them You Care

It's the simple stuff to bring profitability.

The docs who don't care about their patients have disloyal patients.
The docs who care about their patients have fiercely loyal patients.

Don't give me the eye roll. I have had this conversation so many times I'm immune to it. Oh, I know. There are a few doctors out there who don't care but have made money.

But what I know is the docs who care have enduring careers and profitable practices.

Storytime…

How many of you are in charge of the practice during weekend hours? You know what I mean. It is Saturday night, 8pm, and you are in charge of taking the calls/old school pager/or whatever system you have to hear from patients if they have an eye emergency. And I know you have gone into the office a dozen times for an "emergency" that turned out to be an eyelash stuck in someone's eye. But to the tale.

This one doctor owned the practice outright. It was him and him alone. So, every phone call was his. There was a period of time when he answered the call with the desire to serve well. And like any of you, he also had to talk himself into an eagerness to serve as he opened the door.

But over time, he couldn't talk himself into eagerness anymore.

Now, a small percentage of your patients see you after hours, so what does it matter if you aren't the friendliest to one here or there? What does it matter if you don't convince one or two of them you care? You opened up night, right?

Well, not caring caught up to this doctor.

He showed up to care for the patient, but he wasn't in a good mood, and the patient could tell. It was a scratched cornea, which is treated easily, so he cared for the patient and scheduled her for the following Monday.

Well, she returned Monday with her husband..and he wasn't happy.

The doctor protested. He came in on a weekend. Her cornea was better. Why were they mad?

But none of that changed the husband's opinion. Yes, the doctor came in on a weekend and took care of her cornea. But those things were not enough to convince the patient (or her husband) that he cared.

So, the eye got better, and the patients left. No big deal, right?

But, just like we talked about in providing quality eye care, you care for your patients, and they refer. You don't care for your patients, and they tell a dozen people how you don't care for the people you see.

I'm not asking you to fake caring for you patients. I don't think you can. I'm asking you to care for patients so well that you convince them that you enjoy caring for them.

Listen, I want you to have good systems. I want you to have a great front desk person. But if you don't care for patients, you might eek by a profit. Growing profitability is going to take caring for patients, and it is going to take their believing it more than anything else.

You will increase revenue if your patents trust you care for them.

Spiff Your Staff

I wholeheartedly believe in the final element of increasing revenues.

No matter how great of a staff you have, no matter how conscientious they may be, not matter how loyal they have been to you, they still need to be motivated.

And I'm afraid the largest, most enduring motivation is to make more money. This is why I told the story at the beginning of the book. I took pride in my job. I liked doing it well. But when my doctor gave me the motivation of a percentage of net profits, I upped my game. I cared about the paperclips.

You may have the best frame seller in the world, but when you tell them they can get an extra hundred bucks if they sell 40 frames in a month (or however many you choose per your 2.5 turnover a month calculation), they will sell like crazy.

Now, I want to give you a couple of options for how you can spiff (bonus) your staff. So, let's start with the frame seller.

Let's say you have 400 frames on your board.
400 X 2.5 = 1,000 frames you need to sell a year.
You are open 5 days a week for 52 weeks, so that's 260 business days.
1,000 frames divided by 260 business days = roughly 4 frames a day.
1,000 frames divided by 52 weeks = roughly 20 frames a week.

Now, this is not a lot of frames. 400 frames on a frame board is not a huge board, but you can figure out the numbers for yourself.

But let's use the numbers above for our example.

4 frames a day is not a ton. It's not. So, up your frame seller's game. You know you need 20 frames a week or 80 or so a month. So, you spiff your frame seller on 5 frames a day, 25 a month, or 100 a month. Here's the thing though: make sure that the average you are spiffing them on is above the average that they were already selling.

And what does the frame seller get if they sell 100 frames a month? $100.

Now, don't worry about the $100. If they sell an extra frame a day, an extra 20 a month, you are making a ton more money. I'm assuming your profit on a frame sell (just the frame sell alone, I'm not even talking the lens), is probably $100 per frame.

Your seller sells an extra 20 frames per month, with a $100 profit per, you are making an extra $2,000 a month. You give the seller a $100, and you net an extra $1,900.

Then, create a spiff for every position in your office. Just make sure every spiff is based on, either an improvement from that position's average, or based above what you need the office to do.

Does your front desk keep the schedule 90% full? Spiff them on weeks above 95%.

Does your tech sell 50 photos a month? Spiff them on what they sell above 60.

Does your contact lens tech sell 100 year's supply a month? Spiff them on 125.

Then, spiff your entire staff on office goals. That way everybody gets to enjoy some of the fun.

Show the staff what the deposits were for the same month in the prior year. If they increase the deposits by 5%, they get $100 (every one of them). 10% gets them $125, and on and on. Again, you are making more money, and they are more motivated.

Let me show you what this might look like…

You'll see last year's deposit numbers. Then, you project what 5%, 10%, and on would be. You show the staff how much they get if they hit those numbers, and tell them to go for it. You will be amazed at hard they work for these bonuses.

Last Yr.	Dep	5% ($100)	10% ($125)	15% ($150)	20% ($175)
Jan	66,327	69,643	72,960	76,276	79,592
Feb	71,754	75,342	78,929	82,517	86,105
Mar	80,858	84,901	88,944	92,987	97,030
April	87,763	92,151	96,539	101,042	105,316
May	77,089	80,943	84,798	88,652	92,507
June	80,223	84,234	88,256	92,256	96,268
July	71,673	75,257	78,840	82,424	86,008
Aug	75,674	79,458	83,241	87,025	90,809
Sep	76,026	79,827	83,629	87,430	91,231
Oct	81,950	86,048	90,145	94,143	98,340
Nov	62,457	65,580	68,703	71,826	74,948
Dec	67,525	70,901	74,278	77,654	81,030

Spiffs make for a motivated staff.
A motivated staff creates more revenue.
More revenue leads to more profits (if you have put into place the 3 steps).

Let's answer a few questions.

Questions

Do you have a quality, friendly front desk person? Why or why not?

If you do, what makes them such a good front desk person? If not, why do you still keep them around?

Ask 3 random patients over the course of a day to give you their opinion of your front desk person. Make sure one of them is a new patient. Write down their reactions here.

At what point do you think you exercised the most care for your patients? What characterized that time?

If you are not caring for your patients as well as you once did, what is keeping you from that level of care?

Think of a time recently when you might have cared for your patients better. Think specifically about you could have done better and write them down here. What is your plan to not do that again?

First things first, find out your averages.

What percentage of your schedule is full each month?

How many frames do you need to sell each month to turn your board over 2.5 times a year?

How many photos do you sell in a month?

How many year's supplies of contacts do you sell in a month?

Create a spread sheet with your monthly deposits for each month of last year.

Once you have those numbers, put into place goal deposits for your staff and then have a staff meeting to talk about the new spiffs.

Remember, all spiffs are based on improvement from prior performance. That way you never lose money.

To Sum it Up

So, here we are at the end. The final step towards working towards profitability is increasing revenue.

To increase your revenue, you are going to need to start at your front desk, making sure you have the best, friendliest person making sure your patients are greeted well, cared for, and checked out well.

And your patients have got to believe you care about them. If you have not put the time or effort into them that you once did, then you have got to convince them you do care. Address what in yourself is keeping you from giving the best care. The best cared for patients are your best marketing.

Finally, spiff your employees. Spiff your employees. Spiff 'em. I cannot stress this enough. Even the best staff needs motivation, and money will motivate them more than anything else. As long as their bonus is based on improvement, you will never lose a dollar by spiffing them.

One Final Note

So, that is it, friends. We are at the end.

Do not be discouraged. Caring for people and providing quality eye care is a noble profession. You have been trained well. You know what you are doing.

So, now let's make a profit. Or, let's increase the profit you already make. Follow these 3 steps, and go back over and over to them.

Always provide the best eye care. Remember your oath. Take your time, and hire quality staff

Keep your costs low. Don't overstock. Find the right price point. And manage your frame sellers.

Increase revenues. Start at your front desk. Convince your patients that you care. Spiff your staff.

And if you do those things, you will be way ahead in returning to or increasing your profit.

Thanks for letting me be a part of your practice. Please know that I'm always available to help. I consult in person. I tele-consult. And I organize eye doctor masterminds.

Just email me at jgordonduncan@gmail.com if you would like to find out how I might help more. Additionaly, if you email me, I will be glad to give you references of doctors that I have helped. I can give you cell phone numbers of doctors who would be glad to speak to you directly.

Talk to you soon.

Gordon Duncan

E-books from Gordon Duncan and Jobson Research

<u>Practice Progress - How to Maximize Eye Care Revenue</u>

This is no mere book. It is a toolkit to enable you to increase your Optometric Revenue. Practice Progress works like this. In it, you'll learn diagnostic tools to enable you to determine the health of your Optometric practice.

You will hear about incentive programs that motivate staff. Formulas and examples will be provided to help you and your staff project how healthy a month is going to be, and then practical tips will be provided to enable you to improve those results.

The end goal is that your practice will begin practicing the progress you want it to make.

<u>TeleTivoNetting: Accomplishing More by Doing Less</u>

Isn't it ironic that most time-efficiency systems come in books that are 300 pages long? Well, TeleTivoNetting hopes to counter that. Less words...more productivity.

The idea is accomplishing more by doing less. This 3-Step process is easy to understand and easy to implement.

TeleTivoNetting will explain each step, give you both successful and failed examples, and even give you opportunities to help examine areas of your life and practice.

Hopefully, when you are done, you will be armed with a system that will help you and your office be more productive and even more restful.

Simple. Enjoy.

Which is Better: One or Two? Improving the Vision of Your Practice

The eye industry is being challenged. In fact, it might be in its most challenging age yet. Salary demands are climbing, but quality staff are diminishing. Governmental insurance demands make it more difficult to collect and make money. Specialized skills like filing insurance, selling frames, and understanding the science of optics are becoming harder to find. More and more Optometrists are graduating from school. There are less and less jobs. Oh, by the way, did I mention that many of these graduates have over $100,000 in school debt? Optometrists nearing retirement are finding it difficult to find younger OD's who can afford to buy their practices. It is not uncommon for a practice to have six figures in outstanding insurance. The bottom line is that Optometrists are just plain old tired. And while no single book is going to address or solve are these problems, this small book is intended to encourage you to enjoy the industry once again. To get you there, to help you enjoy walking in your office again, we are going to take an approach with which you are incredibly familiar. Just like you ask your patients, I'm going to ask you:

Which is better: One or Two?
What you'll find in the following chapters is three specific areas that if you apply the one or two model, you'll find an enjoyment in your practice, you'll find enjoyment with your staff, and you'll find enjoyment with your patients.

So, without any more waiting, here are your questions.
Which is Better: One or Two?
Whose Glory are You Seeking? Yours or the Practice's?
Who Has to Be Right? You or the Best Idea?
What are You Zealous for? Profits or Patients?
Let's tackle these one by one, and along the way, we'll work through both good and bad examples. Then we'll find give you an opportunity to work through the "one or two" yourself.

Enjoy.

About the Author

Author, Gordon Duncan, is an award-winning educator, salesman, teacher, manager, and writer.

He has taught in the public school system, lobbied for schools' accreditations, managed eye clinics, led sales' teams, run marathons, and even published a book on theology.

He has been happily married to Amy for over 20 years and is the proud father of 3 wonderful girls.

You can find more about him at almost all social media platforms. If you would like to know more day to day about his thoughts on optometry, find him at

fb.me/optometricrescue

and…

https://www.instagram.com/od_rescue/

And of course, you can always email him at jgordonduncan@gmail.com.